Use of Propranolol for Stress
The Long View
Your 21st Psychiatric Consultation
William R. Yee M.D., J.D.,
Copyright Applied for Jan. 30, 2021

Propranolol is a medication that blocks adrenaline.

Adrenaline is a hormone that is released by stress which causes an increase in heart rate, muscle strength, blood pressure, and sugar metabolism.

Adrenaline is believed to be part of a physiologic survival strategy that prepares the individual for "flight or fight" over millions of years of adaptation to a hunter gatherer lifestyle.

However, the adrenaline based "flight or fight" response is an inherited maladaptation to post hunter gatherer societies.

Stressors in the modern world are not temporary and solved by flight or fight.

In the modern world the individual goes to work on a regular basis to spend eight or more hours a day in a stressful environment.

The modern work environment is designed to continually increase productivity.

In the modern world MBA's continually find ways to increase productivity.

This results in a work environment where the worker is faced with stress and the knowledge that the stress will increase in the future.

Many workers have the hopeless feeling and belief that the productivity standards will increase until they fail.

The employer and the MBA's know that as the productivity standards increase, the percentage of workers that fail will increase.

That is not a problem for the employer and the MBA because the workers that fail will leave and the burden of retirement benefits for the corporation will diminish.

The employer's view is often that workers are not valued employees and assets, but rather disposable commodities on the labor market.

The stress can increase to the point that the workers die from the stress.

The Japanese have a word for this, Karoshi. The literal translation of Karoshi is "death by overwork"

Karoshi: Is It Sweeping America?
 Conway, Mara Eleina
Publication Date 1997
Journal Pacific Basin Law Journal, 15(2)
UCLA Pacific Basin Law Journal
Peer reviewed
https://escholarship.org/uc/item/2v29n6v0

Takotsubo Syndrome is a sudden and acute form of heart failure. Symptoms can be similar to a heart attack. It is also known as Takotsubo Cardiomyopathy, Broken Heart Syndrome, Acute Stress Induced Cardiomyopathy, Apical

Ballooning, Acute Stress-Induced Cardiomyopathy, Takotsubo Syndrome, or just Takotsubo for short.

It's not known exactly what causes Takotsubo, but it's often brought on by emotional or physical distress. Some examples of triggers may include:
1. bereavement
2. domestic abuse
3. physical assault
4. acute illness
5. recent surgery
6. financial worries or debt
7. being involved in a disaster, such as an earthquake.

High levels of Catecholamines cause:
1. high blood pressure
2. heart palpitations
3. anxiety
4. shaking
5. excessive sweating
6. pale skin
7. tingling in the fingers and toes
8. blurred vision
9. severe headaches
10. abdominal pain
11. sickness

12. constipation
13. weight loss
14. high blood sugar
15. psychiatric disturbances

Catecholamines cause intracellular Ca2+ overload, coronary spasm, myocardial cell damage, depletion of high energy stores, ventricular arrhythmias, and sudden cardiac death.
See:
Role of catecholamine oxidation in sudden cardiac death
Naranjan S Dhalla 1, Adriana Adameova, Meera Kaur
Affiliations expand
Fundam Clin Pharmacol. 2010 Oct;24(5):539-46. doi: 10.1111/j.1472-8206.2010.00836.x.
PMID: 20584205 DOI: 10.1111/j.1472-8206.2010.00836.x

It is appropriate to test for catecholamines which may reach the extraordinarily high level of 35.9 ng/ml in acute stress.
See:
Role of the excessive amounts of circulating catecholamines and

glucocorticoids in stress-induced heart disease

Adriana Adameova 1, Yasser Abdellatif, Naranjan S Dhalla

PMID: 19767873 DOI: 10.1139/y09-042

Propranolol/Inderal may be used to treat:
angina pectoris,
hypertension,
cardiac arrhythmias,
myocardial infarction,
essential hypertension,
treatment of resistant arterial hypertension,
migraine headaches,
essential tremors,
anxiety disorders, target symptoms being:
8. autonomic,
9. hyperactivity,
10. hyperarousal
GAD (Generalized Anxiety Disorder), target symptoms being:
11. tachycardia,
12. palpitations,
13. sweating, and
14. tremors.
Performance Anxiety (Stage Fright)
PTSD

15. Unpleasant Memories, it has an amnestic effect in PTSD
16. Improves cognitive function which aids psychotherapy of PTSD

Portal Hypertension
Hyperthyroidism
Pheochromocytoma
Drug Craving in drug addiction
Stress of newly diagnosed cancer

Because there are so many uses for propranolol, it is often used in the context of asthma which is a relative contraindication for propranolol.

"Propranolol is generally well tolerated. Common adverse events include gastrointestinal disturbances, bradycardia, hypotension, bronchospasm, exertional dyspnea, hypoglycemia, dizziness, fatigue, and insomnia. These are usually mild and can be managed conservatively without requiring discontinuation of medication. Further, propranolol has demonstrated safety for use in pediatric patients."

See:

Propranolol: A 50-Year Historical
Perspective
A. V. Srinivasan

Ann Indian Acad Neurol. 2019 Jan-Mar;
22(1): 21–26.
doi: 10.4103/aian.AIAN_201_18
PMCID: PMC6327687
PMID: 30692755

I have been practicing medicine for about
fifty years and I have been prescribing
propranolol, also known as Inderal for
about fifty years.

During those fifty years I have not had a
single patient die of any medication I
prescribed except for one patient.

That patient was taking lithium that I
prescribed in a nursing home.

The patient that died from the lithium I
prescribed was an elderly lady who
developed pneumonia.

She, like many other elderly people, had a
silent pneumonia without symptoms.

She simply slept.

When the staff realized that she had pneumonia they called me.

I ordered that the lithium be stopped, and I ordered a stat lithium level.

It was very high.

It was too late.

She died of lithium toxicity.

You never forget the first and only patient that died due to side effects of a medication you prescribe.

I am here to do no harm and help if I can.

Thank you for your time and attention.

William R. Yee M.D., J.D.
Board Certified Psychiatrist.
Practicing Medicine and Psychiatry without
interruption since 1972 in Michigan, Indiana,
Kentucky, California and Texas.

Recently licensed in Texas and excited about
opportunities to live and practice in Texas, at
your service.

"Pre-Existing text," includes names of symptoms, medical illnesses, medications, people, corporations, law cases, statutes, text of statutes, the titles of articles, titles of books, the content of articles and books cited.

My copyright claim is a clam to the "original text," which is my personal experiences as
described in the text above, and my commentary on the names of symptoms, medical illnesses, medications, people, corporations, law cases, statues, text of statutes, the titles of articles, of books, the content of articles and books cited.

Depression, Anxiety, Anger, and
Behaviors, The Long View
Your 23rd Psychiatric Consultation
William R. Yee M.D., J.D.
Copyright Applied for March 20th, 2021

I started treating anxiety, depression,
anger, and behavior disorders in 1972.

At the first visit I educate the patient on
the management of symptoms of mental
illness, medications, and psychiatric
treatment in general.

I then offer the patient the options to
choose from the following list of
medications:

Propranolol for stress, anxiety and panic
attacks.
Prazosin for nightmares, anxiety and
panic attacks.
Buspirone for anxiety.
Escitalopram for anxiety, depression,
panic attacks and low energy.
Mirtazapine for anxiety, depression, panic
attacks and insomnia.
Amitriptyline for anxiety, depression,
panic attacks, insomnia and pain.

Chlorpromazine for anxiety, anger, mood swings, paranoia,
hallucinations, mood instability, Bipolar Mania, Schizophrenia and
pain.
There are hundreds of additional medications that may be tried.

I consider these medications to be the safest medications for starting.

Currently when the patient opts for Amitriptyline for anxiety, depression, panic attacks, insomnia and pain I refer them to the pain clinic due to institutional policies, procedures, and practices.

The choice of Amitriptyline is for educational and referral purposes.

The reason I indicate that, "There are hundreds of additional medications that may be tried," is because I let patients know that I am willing to offer medications one at a time until the patient has tried them all, finds a medication that is effective, or decides that medications are a waste of the patient's time and money.

I also offer weekly appointments until the medication is optimized to the best balance of benefits or side effects.

If the patient refuses follow-up appointments, I advise the patient that I am open to additional appointments any time the patient chooses to call and schedule an appointment.

I make a note that future appointments are PRN at the patient's convenience.

It is always the patient's choice as to when the patient sees me.

Treating depression, anxiety, and anger with medications is a simple matter of trying medications, starting with the safest and progressing through the ranks of safety to the most dangerous medications, such as Clozaril which requires weekly blood tests for low white blood cell counts.

Treating Behavior Disorders is another matter.

Nothing is easy in medicine.

Half of emergency room physicians and seven of ten nurses in emergency rooms report that they have been assaulted.

The physical assaults are accompanied by threats and false allegations of abuse at the hands of the physicians and nurses.

I rely on:

Rising violence in the emergency department
Ken Budd, Special to AAMCNews
February 24, 2020

Behavior Disorders require the patient to change.

The psychologist, social worker, and psychiatrist cannot force a patient to change.

The psychologist, social worker, psychiatrist can educate the patient as to the benefits of change.

The psychologist, social worker, psychiatrist can educate the patient as to the adverse effects of not changing.

The psychologist, social worker, psychiatrist can give the patient tools to change such as:

1. Education as to sleep hygiene
2. Education as to meditation
3. Education as to sleep diaries
4. Education as to symptom and medication diaries
5. Education as to deep breathing
6. Education as to relaxation techniques
7. Education as to symptom substitution, finger snapping to replace hair pulling etc.

The patient, however, must change and the health care worker cannot force the change.

The health care worker may use Cognitive Behavior Therapy to accelerate the rate of change, but the patient must make the decision to change. That decision is evidenced by change.

Behavior disorders are a choice the patient makes, and the patient must change the choice.

Now the reader must understand the concept of resistance to treatment.

Why does the patient persist in behaviors that create obesity, drug addiction, self-mutilation, gambling, credit card spending, knowing that it causes more harm than good?

Good question, the answer and cure to that question is a Nobel Prize in Medicine.

We now have an epidemic of obesity and all its adverse effects including diabetes and death.

We now have an epidemic of drug addiction that is worse than it was in 1972 when I started practicing medicine.

Prohibition did not solve the problem of alcoholism, and merely bankrolled Al Capone and Organized Crime.

I have prescribed Antabuse (Disulfiram) and patients have told me that they drank alcohol while using Antabuse. Antabuse causes a toxic effect with alcohol that is very unpleasant and can be lethal. The use of Antabuse is based upon negative reinforcement. Instead of euphoria from alcohol the patient suffers horribly.

The FDA has given approval for three drugs for the treatment of alcoholism:
Antabuse (Disulfiram) as a Drinking Deterrent
Naltrexone for Alcohol Cravings
Campral (Acamprosate) for Discomfort

Even though these three drugs have been around for years, they have not had a substantial impact on the rate of alcoholism. Their impact on addiction is only marginally greater than the placebo effect.

I rely on:
Pharmacotherapy of Alcohol Use
Disorders: Seventy-Five Years of Progress
Leah R. Zindel, R.PH., M. A. L. Sa and
Henry R. Kranzler, M.D.
J Stud Alcohol Drugs Suppl. 2014 Mar;
75(Suppl 17): 79–88.
PMCID: PMC4453501
PMID: 24565314

and
Pharmacological treatments for opiate
and alcohol addiction: A historical
perspective of the last 50 years
M. Carmen Blanco-Gandía, Marta
Rodríguez-Arias
Publication: European Journal of
Pharmacology
European Journal of Pharmacology
Volume 836, 5 October 2018, Pages 89-101

My experience with behavior disorders is
that the patients have had the behavior
for years before meeting me. Most often
their behaviors emerged in childhood and
adolescence as oppositional defiant
disorders, conduct disorders, borderline
personality disorders, antisocial

personality disorders and substance use disorders among other disorders.

The behavior disorders affect ability to function in the family, school, community and work.

By the time the patient arrives in the office the common sense changes that I recommend have already been offered by parents, siblings, teachers, spouses and employers and rejected by the patient.

Very often the patient will respond with the same tools that the patient used with parents, siblings, teachers, spouses and employees.

The patient will attempt to recruit the mental health worker as a codependent in blaming parents, siblings, teachers, spouses and employees for the patient's behaviors.

The patient often gives an unreliable history.

Memory is not reliable and easily
influenced by the technique used for
interrogation.

I rely on
The fallibility of memory in judicial
processes: Lessons from the past and their
modern consequences
Mark L. Howe, and Lauren M. Knott
Memory. 2015 Jul 4; 23(5): 633–656.
Published online 2015 Feb 23. doi:
10.1080/09658211.2015.1010709
PMCID: PMC4409058
PMID: 25706242

Borderline Personality Disorder emerged
in the early 1970's from studies of
treatment failures in psychiatry.

After the known mental illnesses were
eliminated, a pool of treatment failures
was sorted out by factor analytic
strategies and a group was isolated with
common symptoms and given the label
Borderline Personality Disorder.

This group was originally isolated from a
pool of treatment failures after all the
known treatments had failed.

This group continues to crowd mental health centers, hospital emergency rooms and psychiatric hospitals despite interventions by multiple psychiatrists, multiple medications, and multiple intervention strategies. They remain largely refractory to treatment.

Neurocognitive deficits may be the root cause of Borderline Personality Disorder and explain the pervasive failure of medications and psychotherapies in providing significant remission of symptoms.

I rely on

Borderline personality disorder and neuropsychological measures of executive function: A systematic review
Personality and Mental Health 10(1)
September 2015
DOI: 10.1002/pmh.1320

Borderline Personality Disorders typically are field dependent rather than field independent in thinking and behavior.

Their thinking and behavior change radically in the presence of different people and different situations.

This is related to their lack of boundaries.

This explains the disparity of clinical presentation during the same day in the presence of different behavioral health specialists.

Borderline Personality Disorder is identified by the following stigmata:

1. identity diffusion
2. interpersonal disturbances
3. chronic instability
4. episodes of extreme affective states
5. loss of control of impulses
6. field dependent behavior

I rely on

Early Detection and Outcome in Borderline Personality Disorder
Paola Bozzatello, Silvio Bellino†, Marco Bosia and Paola Rocca
Front. Psychiatry, 09 October 2019 | https://doi.org/10.3389/fpsyt.2019.00710

Attention deficit hyperactivity disorder (ADHD) is a developmental disorder, identified by the presence of

8. Hyperactivity
9. Impulsivity
10. Inattention.

ADHD is identified in 2.5% of the population and manifests with:

11. cognitive impairments
12. emotional impairments
13. social functioning impairments
14. activity of daily living impairments.

I rely on

Driving and Road Rage Associated with Attention Deficit Hyperactivity Disorder (ADHD): a Systematic Review.
Deshmukh, P., Patel, D.
Curr Dev Disord Rep 6, 241–247 (2019).
https://doi.org/10.1007/s40474-019-00183-9
Published 07 November 2019
Issue Date December 2019
DOIhttps://doi.org/10.1007/s40474-019-00183-9

Complex tasks such as driving, flying an airplane or entry into hostage situations in a bank robbery gone wrong involve but are not limited to:

1. vigilance
2. focus
3. impulse control
4. rapid integration of complex data sets
5. rapid decision making
6. integration of complex frontal lobe executive
    functions
7. memory
8. visuospatial functions
9. executive control of emotional state
10. mature personality traits often
    referred to as parenting or superego
     functions

Attention Deficit Disorder manifests with:
1. inattention, an impairment
2. impulsivity, an impairment
3. executive dysfunction, an impairment
4. selective attention impairment
5. divided attention impairment
6. flexibility/set shifting impairment
7. vigilance/sustained attention impairment

8. working memory impairment
9. impulse control impairment
10. fluency functions impairment
11. planning and problem-solving impairment
12. concept formation impairment
13. cognitive flexibility impairment
14. social cognition impairment
15. time perception impairment

I rely on:
Driving and attention deficit hyperactivity disorder

Anselm B. M. Fuermaier, Lara Tucha, Ben Lewis Evans, Janneke Koerts, Dick de Waard, Karel Brookhuis, Steffen Aschenbrenner, Johannes Thome, Klaus W. Lange, and Oliver Tucha1
J Neural Transm (Vienna). 2017; 124(Suppl 1): 55–67.
Published online 2015 Sep 29. doi: 10.1007/s00702-015-1465-6
PMCID: PMC5281661
PMID: 26419597

ADHD and criminal behavior are issues I confronted during many years of work in prisons since 1987.

Between a fourth and a third of juvenile and adult prisoners suffer from ADHD.

What does this mean to employers and social groups attempting to integrate ADHD into their ranks?

Employees with ADHD display nonconforming behavior and the disruption of rules and organizational structure including but not limited to:

1. inconsistent attendance
2. failure to complete tasks,
3. inability to stay on assigned tasks
4. irritability and hostility to supervisors
5. violation of institutional rules
6. poor judgment in execution of assigned tasks
7. unsafe operation of police vehicle
8. unsafe use of weapons during civil unrest
9. unsafe use of weapons during hostage situations
10. shooting innocent bystanders impulsively
11. shooting other police officers impulsively

Primary missions for police agencies in this country include managing civil unrest and hostage situations.

The fact that one quarter to one third of juvenile and adult prisoners have ADHD is is a red flag for police agencies hiring and training in police academies.

There should be a screening of new recruits because impairment in the safe use and operation of police vehicles in high-speed chase and the use of guns and other weapons in civil unrest and hostage situations is not an acceptable risk for public safety.

In addition, impairment of frontal lobe executive functions and inability to recognize and conform to rules of social conduct is disruptive to the orderly operation of the police agency.

Public Safety is a huge issue that police agencies across the country are facing and there is a great deal of controversy including the extreme solution of defunding police.

I rely on:

A meta-analysis of the prevalence of attention deficit hyperactivity disorder in incarcerated populations
S. Young, D. Moss, O. Sedgwick, M. Fridman, and P. Hodgkins
Psychol Med. 2015 Jan; 45(2): 247–258.
Published online 2014 Apr 7. doi: 10.1017/S0033291714000762
PMCID: PMC4301200
PMID: 25066071

Police Agencies should be investing in tests that identify impulsivity and other issues in the safe use of guns. They should not rely on questionnaires and subjective reporting and subjective observation. They should be using computer programs that do not allow for manipulation of data by the subject.

P-drive, and TRIP were identified as highly qualified on-road driving tests. Future studies should confirm measurement error, content validity, structural validity, responsiveness, and interpretability of these tools.

I rely on
Standardized on-road tests assessing fitness-to-drive in people with cognitive impairments: A systematic review
David Bellagamba,
Line Vionnet,
Isabel Margot-Cattin,
Paul Vaucher
Published: May 18, 2020
https://doi.org/10.1371/journal.pone.0233125

and
A Systematic Review and Meta-Analysis of On-Road Simulator and Cognitive Driving Assessment in Alzheimer's Disease and Mild Cognitive Impairment
Megan A Hird 1 2, Peter Egeto 3, Corinne E Fischer 1 4, Gary Naglie 5 6 7, Tom A Schweizer 1 8 9
J Alzheimers Dis. 2016 May 11;53(2):713-29. doi: 10.3233/JAD-160276.
PMID: 27176076 DOI: 10.3233/JAD-160276

Human factors, as opposed to vehicle and environmental factors are the primary cause of automobile accidents.

Human factors are also the most likely root cause of police officers shooting innocent bystanders and other police officers in hostage situations and during civil unrest.

In high income countries motor vehicle accidents are the primary cause of death among children, adolescents, and adults to the age of 29.

Accidents account for more than two-thirds of all injuries.

The root cause of accidents and errors in the use of guns and weapons used in hostage situations and civil unrest is impaired executive functioning.

ADHD manifests impaired executive functioning with
    15. inattention
    16. Impulsiveness
    17. Hyperactivity
    18. risk taking.

19. Speeding
20. following too close
21. driving under the influence of alcohol
22. cell phone use
23. not using seatbelts
24. personality traits including risk taking
25. sensation seeking
26. difficulty in dealing with tension
27. difficulty in dealing controlling anger
28. substance abuse
29. antisocial tendencies
30. non-conformity
31. risky driving behaviors
32. low parental involvement
33. negative peer and parental influence
34. poor risk perception
35. impaired capacity to deploy appropriate judgment and reasoning

I rely on

What We Know About ADHD and Driving Risk: A Literature Review, Meta-Analysis and Critique

Laurence Jerome, MB. Ch.B., M.Sc.,
M.R.C., Psych., F.R.C.P.C.(C), Alvin Segal,
Ph.D., and Liat Habinski, B.Sc.
PMCID: PMC2277254
PMID: 18392181

Police work, use of police cars, guns and
weapons during civil unrest can result in
heavy tolls on police departments and
police officers.

Stress in Police Work has root causes in:
1. shift work
2. work interfering with home life,
3. lack of consultation with supervisors
4. lack of communication with supervisors
5. lack of control over workload
6. inadequate support from the employer
7. excess workload
8. organizational culture

I rely on:
Stress in police officers: a study of the
origins, prevalence and severity of stress-
related symptoms within a county police
force
P. A. Collins, A. C. C. Gibbs

Occupational Medicine, Volume 53, Issue
4, June 2003, Pages 256–264,
https://doi.org/10.1093/occmed/kqg061
Published: 01 June 2003

and
Shift Work and Occupational Stress in
Police Officers
Claudia C. Ma1Michael E. Andrew, Desta
Fekedulegn, Ja K. Gu, Tara, A. Hartley,
Luenda E. Charles, John M. Violanti, Cecil
M. Burchfiel
Safety and Health at Work
Volume 6, Issue 1, March 2015, Pages 25-29

Stress in Police Work can be
overwhelming with many adverse
outcomes including:
1. prior diagnosis of mental illness
2. depression
3. anxiety
4, PTSD
5. suicidal ideation
6. self-harm symptom
7. suicide

I rely on:
Prevalence of Mental Illness and Mental
Health Care Use Among Police Officers

Katelyn K. Jetelina, MPH, PhD; Rebecca
J. Molsberry, MPH; Jennifer Reingle
Gonzalez, MS, PhD2; et al; Alaina M.
Beauchamp, MPH; Trina Hall, PhD.
JAMA Netw Open. 2020;3(10):e2019658.
October 7, 2020
doi:10.1001/jamanetworkopen.2020.19658

Anxiety Disorders are associated with
structural and functional changes in the
brain that affect:
1. the hippocampus
2. anterior cingulate cortex and amygdala,
3. impairs functional connectivity in the
central
    executive network
4. nodes in the sensorimotor network
5. pre- and postcentral volume, reduced
6. supplementary motor area volume,
7. reduced functional connectivity in
    anterior and posterior cerebellum.

Anxiety Disorders manifest with:
1. irritability
2. difficulty concentrating
3. insomnia
4. fatigue
5. restlessness
6. muscle tension

Before diagnosing and treating ADHD and insomnia in high stress environments such as police organizations the psychiatrist is advised to diagnose and treat stress and anxiety.

I rely on
Systematic review and meta-analyses of neural structural and functional differences in generalized anxiety disorder and healthy controls using magnetic resonance imaging
Tiffany A. Kolesar, Elena Bilevicius, Alyssia D. Wilson, and Jennifer Kornelsena,
Neuroimage Clin. 2019; 24: 102016.
Published online 2019 Oct 14. doi:
10.1016/j.nicl.2019.102016
PMCID: PMC6879983
PMID: 31835287

Stress and anxiety manifest with insomnia, hyperactivity impaired attention and impaired memory that can look like ADHD but remits with treatment of anxiety.

Depression can be agitated and present with impaired attention and memory.

Depression and anxiety should be treated in high stress environments such as police work before ADHD is diagnosed and treated.

This missive is intended to be an introduction to a large and complex topic with sufficient references to upon a window for further research for the serious student, attorney or patient wishing to know more.

It must end at some point, and I will end it here and now.

I am here to do no harm and help if I can.

Thank you for your time and attention.
William R. Yee M.D., J.D.
Board Certified Psychiatrist.
Practicing Medicine and Psychiatry without interruption since 1972 in Michigan, Indiana, Kentucky, California, and Texas, at your service.

"Pre-Existing text," includes names of symptoms, medical illnesses, medications, people, corporations, agencies, law cases, text of law cases, statutes, text of statutes, policies, the text of policies, the titles of articles, of books, the content of articles and books cited.

My copyright claim is a clam to the "original text," which is my personal experiences as described in the text above and my commentary on the names of symptoms,
medical illnesses, medications, people, names of agencies, corporations, law cases, text of law cases, statutes, text of statutes, policies, the text of policies, the titles of articles, of books, the content of articles and books cited.